ENDOMORPH DIET COOKBOOK

WHITLEY SMITH

Copyright ©2020

TABLE OF CONTENT

INTRODUCTION

This book is committed to assisting endomorphs in achieving their fitness, weight loss, and health objectives. Endomorphs frequently struggles more with weight loss than other body types since they have slower metabolisms and higher body fat percentages.

This cookbook was created especially for endomorphs in order to assist them in preparing wholesome meals that would assist their weight loss and wellness objectives.

For endomorphs particularly, we have gathered some of the tastiest and healthiest meals. There are many alternatives available, ranging from quick snacks to hearty dinners and even some delectable desserts. Also, each meal provides information on calories and macronutrients so you can be sure you're consuming the proper ratio of nutrients.

So, if you're an endomorph looking to lose weight, gain muscle, and live a healthier lifestyle, this cookbook is the perfect place to start.

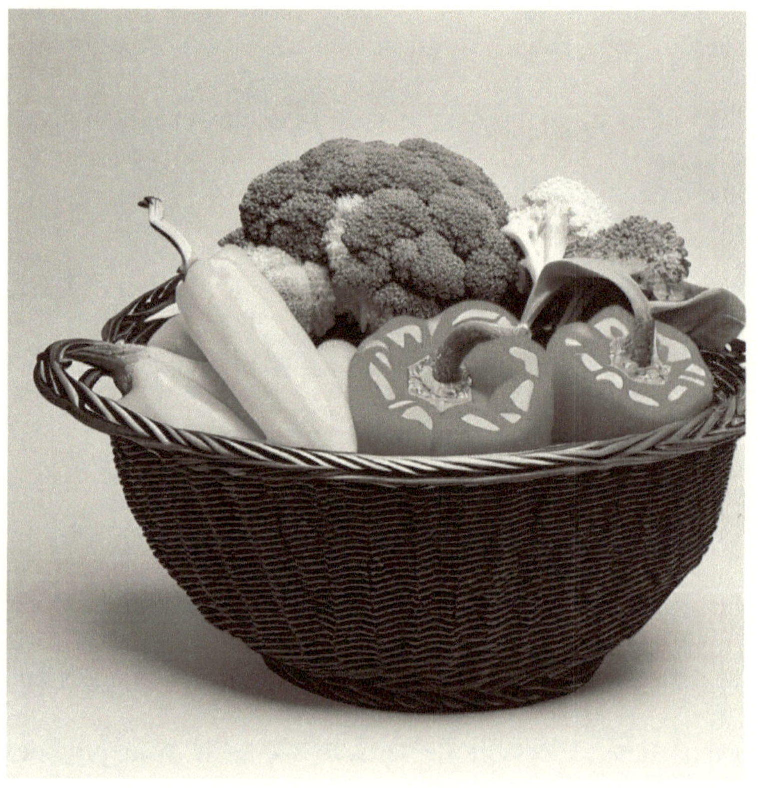

CHAPTER ONE

Understanding the Endomorph Body Type

An endomorph is a body type characterized by a high amount of body fat, round bones, and difficulty adding muscular mass. Endomorphs frequently have higher body fat percentages than average, which can make it challenging to reduce weight and put on muscle.

Moreover, endomorphs frequently have shorter limbs and smaller total stature. Exercises that requires endurance, like swimming, jogging, and cycling, are great for endomorphs since they help them burn fat and develop muscle. Endomorphs should concentrate on maintaining a balanced diet that includes plenty of fresh produce, lean meats, and healthy fats. In addition, they should be sure to get enough rest and refrain from overtraining. Endomorphs can attain their fitness goals and feel and look their best with the right diet and activity.

Endomorphs should remember that their physical characteristics are not a barrier to achieving their goals, but rather a chance to determine the best workout and dietary regimen for them.

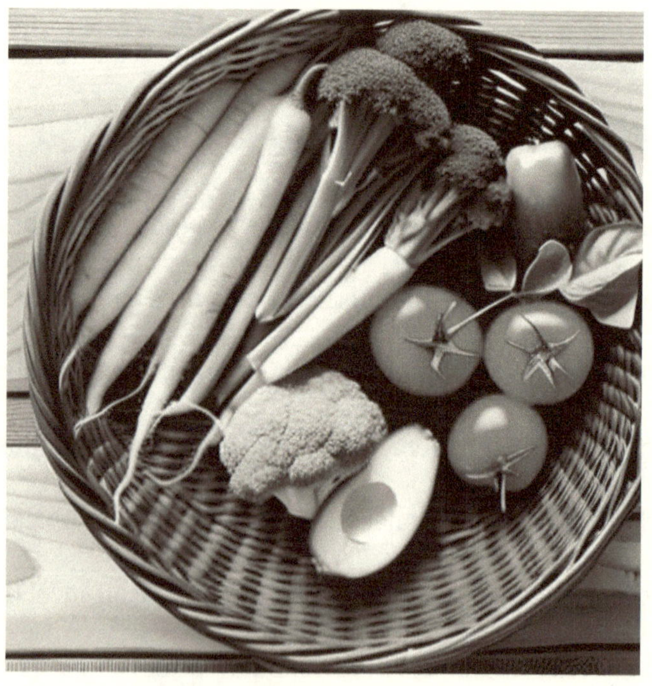

CHAPTER TWO

Essential Nutrients for the Endomorph Diet

Protein

In order to maintain good body composition, protein is a crucial macronutrient for endomorphs because it promotes the growth and maintenance of muscle mass. Protein is essential for a strong immune system and for supplying the body with energy during physical activity. Lean meats, dairy products, eggs, beans, legumes, nuts, and seeds are all good sources of protein for endomorphs.

Complex Carbohydrates

Energy for endomorphs primarily comes from complex carbohydrates. They are also required for healthy development and growth. Whole grains, vegetables, legumes, nuts, and fruit are all sources of complex carbs.

Healthy Fats

Healthy fats are crucial for endomorphs because they promote healthy cell membranes, and enhance hormone function, and energy. Olive oil, almonds, avocados, and fatty seafood are examples of healthy fats. At least 20–30% of your daily caloric intake should come from healthy fats.

Fibre

Fibre is a crucial ingredient for endomorphs because it supports satiety, regulates blood sugar levels, and keeps the digestive system functioning properly. Whole grains, fruits, vegetables, legumes, nuts, and legume products are all sources of fibre. Strive for at least 25 to 30 grams of fibre per day.

Vitamins and Minerals

In order to maintain healthy metabolism, growth, and development, vitamins and minerals are crucial for endomorphs. Fruits, vegetables, whole grains, legumes, nuts, and seeds are some of the foods that are high in vitamins and minerals. Endomorphs ought to make an effort to eat a range of these things each day.

Water

Endomorphs need water to stay healthy and hydrated, which is why it is so important. Endomorphs should try to consume eight glasses of water or more each day.

Note

Endomorphs should adopt healthy lifestyle practices including getting enough sleep, working out frequently, and stress management. These behaviors will maintain a healthy body balance and aid to improve overall health.

CHAPTER THREE

Endomorph Meal Plan

DAY 1

Breakfast: Overnight Oats

Lunch: Quinoa

Dinner: Mushroom and Black Beans

Snacks: Apple Slices with Peanut Butter

DAY 2

Breakfast: Avocado Toast

Lunch: Mediterranean Salmon Salad

Dinner: Rosemary Citrus and Baked Salmon

Snacks: Avocado Cucumber Bites

DAY 3

Breakfast: Greek Yogurt Parfait

Lunch: Chicken and Broccoli Stir-Fry

Dinner: Beef and Barley Stew

Snacks: Banana Oatmeal Pancakes

DAY 4

Breakfast: Tofu Scramble

Lunch: Tuna Salad

Dinner: Greek Chicken and Farro Salad

Snacks: Baked Pears with Walnuts

DAY 5

Breakfast: Cottage Cheese and Fruit Bowl

Lunch: Turkey and Quinoa Stuffed Peppers

Dinner: Lentil and Kale Soup

Snacks: Baked Apples

DAY 6

Breakfast: Egg and Cheese Burrito

Lunch: Veggie Burrito Bowl

Dinner: Grilled Chicken with Roasted Vegetables

Snacks: Baked Sweet Potato Fries

DAY 7

Breakfast: Turkey Sausage and Egg Wrap

Lunch: Grilled Basil Chicken and Zucchini

Dinner: Red Curry Shrimps and Cilantro Rice

Snacks: Trail Mix

CHAPTER FOUR

ENDOMORPH DIET RECIPES

Breakfast

Overnight Oats

Ingredients

- ✓ ½ cup rolled oats

- ✓ ½ cup unsweetened almond milk

- ✓ ½ tsp cinnamon

- ✓ 1 tsp chia seeds

- ✓ ½ sliced banana

Directions

i. Oats, almond milk, cinnamon, chia seeds, and banana slices should all be combined in a container.

ii.   Put the container in the fridge overnight with the lid on.

Time: Overnight

Serving: 1

Nutritional Value

Calories: 280, Carbohydrates: 47g, Fat: 5g, Protein: 9g

Egg and Veggie

Ingredients

- ✓ 1 whole wheat tortilla

- ✓ 2 large eggs

- ✓ ¼ cup diced cooked sweet potato

- ✓ ¼ cup cooked spinach

- ✓ ¼ cup chopped onion

- ✓ ¼ cup shredded cheddar cheese

Directins

i.   A nonstick skillet should be heated to medium-high.

ii.   Pour the eggs and scramble them until cooked properly.

iii. Sauté the spinach, sweet potato, and onion together until the vegetables are soft.

iv.   Add a cooked egg, vegetables, and cheese to a tortilla. Enjoy the burrito after rolling it up.

Time: 10 minutes

Serving: 1

Nutritional Value

Calories: 375, Carbohydrates: 45g, Fat: 10g, Protein: 18g

Avocado Toast

Ingredients

- ✓ 2 slices whole wheat bread

- ✓ ½ avocado

- ✓ ¼ tsp garlic powder

- ✓ ¼ tsp paprika

- ✓ 1 tbsp freshly squeezed lemon juice.

- ✓ ¼ tsp onion powder

Directions

- ✓ In a toaster, toast bread.

- ✓ In a container, mash the avocado and combine it with the paprika, garlic powder, onion powder, and lemon juice.

- ✓ Put the avocado mixture on the toast and eat.

Time: 5 minutes

Serving: 2

Nutritional Value

Calories: 256, Carbohydrates: 19g, Fat: 15g, Protein: 7g

Peanut Butter and Banana Smoothie

Ingredients

- ✓ 1 banana

- ✓ 2 cups unsweetened almond milk

- ✓ 1 tbsp peanut butter

- ✓ ½ tsp chia seeds

Directions

i. Put all ingredients in a blender and process until smooth.

Time: 5 minutes

Serving: 1

Nutritional Value

Calories: 256, Carbohydrates: 27g, Fat: 11g, Protein: 10g

Greek Yogurt Parfait

Ingredients

- ✓ ½ cup plain Greek yogurt

- ✓ ¼ cup raspberries

- ✓ 2 tbsp chopped walnut

- ✓ ¼ cup blueberries

Directions

In a container, put yogurt, blueberries, raspberries, and walnuts. Enjoy.

Time: 5 minutes

Serving: 1

Nutritional Value

Calories: 261, Carbohydrates: 14g, Fat: 14g, Protein: 19g

Breakfast Quinoa

Ingredient

- ✓ ½ cup cooked quinoa

- ✓ ¼ cup cooked black beans

- ✓ ¼ cup salsa

- ✓ ¼ cup plain Greek yogurt

- ✓ ¼ cup chopped red bell pepper

- ✓ ¼ cup shredded cheddar cheese

Directions

i.   A nonstick skillet should be heated to medium.

ii.   Put the Greek yogurt, quinoa, black beans, and salsa, then combine till heated.

iii.   In a bowl, combine the quinoa mixture with the bell pepper and cheese.

Time: 10 minutes

Serving: 1

Nutritional Value

Calories: 358, Carbohydrates: 37g, Fat: 13g, Protein: 20g

Tofu Scramble

Ingredients

- ✓ ¾ cup crumbled firm tofu

- ✓ ¼ cup diced onion

- ✓ ¼ cup diced bell pepper

- ✓ ¼ tsp garlic powder

- ✓ ¼ tsp turmeric

- ✓ ¼ tsp cumin

Directions

i.   A nonstick skillet should be heated to medium-high.

ii. Tofu, onion, and bell pepper should be added and cooked until the vegetables are soft.

iii. Stir in the cumin, turmeric, and garlic powder until the tofu begins to softly brown. Enjoy.

Time: 10 minutes

Serving: 1

Nutritional Value

Calories: 140, Carbohydrates: 9g, Fat: 6g, Protein: 12g

Cottage Cheese and Fruit Bowl

Ingredients

- ✓ ½ cup cottage cheese

- ✓ ¼ cup diced pineapple

- ✓ ¼ cup diced cantaloupe

- ✓ ¼ cup diced mango

- ✓ 2 tbsp chopped walnuts

Directions

i. In a container, add and mix cottage cheese, pineapple, cantaloupe, mango, and walnuts. Enjoy.

Time: 5 minutes

Serving: 1

Nutritional Value

Calories: 280, Carbohydrates: 22g, Fat: 12g, Protein: 21g

Protein Oatmeal

Ingredients

- ✓ ½ cup rolled oats

- ✓ 1 scoop vanilla protein powder

- ✓ ½ cup unsweetened almond milk

- ✓ 1 teaspoon chia seeds

Directions

Oats, almond milk, protein powder, and chia seeds are all mixed in a pot. Cook while stirring often over medium heat until you are sure the oat is properly cooked.

Time: 10 minutes

Serving: 1

Nutritional Value

Calories: 339, Carbohydrates: 39g, Fat: 7g, Protein: 26g

Egg and Cheese Burrito

Ingredients

- ✓ 1 whole wheat tortilla

- ✓ 2 large eggs

- ✓ ¼ cup shredded cheddar cheese

- ✓ ¼ cup cooked black beans

- ✓ ¼ cup diced onion

- ✓ ¼ cup diced bell pepper

Directions

i.   A nonstick skillet should be heated to medium-high.

ii.   Pour in the eggs and fry them until done. Put the onion, beans, and bell pepper and sauté till the veggies are soft.

iii.   Add the cooked egg, vegetables, and cheese to a tortilla.

Time: 10 minutes

Serving: 1

Nutritional Value

Calories: 375, Carbohydrates: 45g, Fat: 10g, Protein: 18g

Coconut Chia Pudding

Ingredients

- ✓ ½ cup unsweetened almond milk

- ✓ ¼ cup chia seeds

- ✓ ¼ cup shredded coconut

✓ ½ tsp vanilla extract

Directions

✓ Mix almond milk, chia seeds, coconut, and vanilla extract in a container.

✓ Close the lid of the container and set it in the fridge all night.

Time: Overnight

Serving: 1

Nutritional Value

Calories: 305, Carbohydrates: 19g, Fat: 17g, Protein: 10g

Turkey Sausage and Egg Wrap

Ingredients

✓ 1 whole wheat wrap

- ✓ ¼ cup shredded cheddar cheese

- ✓ 1 cooked turkey sausage

- ✓ 2 large eggs

- ✓ ¼ cup diced onions

Directions

i. A nonstick skillet should be heated to medium-high. Pour in the eggs and fry them until done. Once the veggies are soft, add the sausage and onion. Wrap up a cooked egg and sausage in it, then add cheese.

ii. Wrap it up and eat it.

Time: 10 minutes

Serving: 1

Nutritional Value

Calories: 384, Carbohydrates: 34g, Fat: 15g, Protein: 22g

Banana Walnut Muffins

Ingredients

- ✓ 1 cup whole wheat flour

- ✓ 1 tsp baking powder

- ✓ ¼ cup diced walnuts

- ✓ ½ tsp baking soda

- ✓ ½ cup mashed banana

- ✓ ½ cup unsweetened almond milk

- ✓ 2 tbsp of honey

Directions

i.   Set oven to 375 degrees.

ii.   Flour, baking soda, and baking powder should all be combined in a container.

iii.   Mix banana, almond milk, and honey in another container.

iv.   Stir till integrated after adding the wet ingredients to the dry ones. Add walnuts and fold.

v.   Pour the batter into a muffin pan that has been greased and bake the muffins until a wooden skewer in the center of one pulls out clean, this should take 15-20 minutes.

Time: 25 minutes

Serving: 12

Nutritional Value

Carbohydrates: 15g, Fat: 3g, Protein: 3g

Lunch

Mediterranean Salmon Salad

Ingredients

- ✓ 4 ounces of wild-caught salmon
- ✓ 2 cups of baby spinach leave
- ✓ ¼ cup of diced cucumber
- ✓ ¼ cup of crumbled feta cheese
- ✓ ¼ cup of chopped tomatoes
- ✓ ¼ cup of black olives
- ✓ 1 tablespoon of olive oil
- ✓ ¼ tsp of sea salt
- ✓ ¼ tsp of black pepper

Directions

i.   Set the oven to 400 °F.

ii.   Season the salmon with salt and pepper and place it on a baking pan.

iii.   For twelve minutes, bake.

iv.   Spinach, cucumber, feta cheese, tomatoes, and olives should all be combined in a big bowl.

v.   Olive oil should be drizzled over the salad and mixed in.

vi.   Place the salad on a platter, then add the grilled salmon on top.

Time: 15 minutes

Servings: 1

Nutritional Value

Calories: 375 Fat: 23g Carbohydrates: 8g Protein:33g

Fiber: 4g Sugar: 3g

Quinoa

Ingredients

- ✓ 1 cup cooked quinoa

- ✓ ¼ cup cooked black beans

- ✓ ¼ cup cooked corn

- ✓ ½ cup diced bell peppers

- ✓ ¼ cup diced red onion

- ✓ 2 tbsp olive oil

- ✓ ¼ tsp sea salt

- ✓ ¼ tsp black pepper

Directions

i.   Quinoa, black beans, corn, bell peppers, and red onion should all be combined in a medium bowl.

ii.   Add salt and pepper, then pour olive oil over the combination.

iii.   Stir everything up thoroughly.

Time: 10 minutes

Servings: 1

Nutritional Value

Calories: 350 Fat: 17g Carbohydrates: 41g Protein: 8g Fiber: 8g Sugar: 4g

Chicken and Broccoli Stir-Fry

Ingredient

- ✓ 4 ounces of boneless, skinless chicken breast

- ✓ 1 cup broccoli florets

- ✓ ¼ cup diced red bell pepper

- ✓ ¼ cup diced yellow onion

- ✓ 1 tbsp of olive oil

- ✓ ¼ tsp of sea salt

- ✓ ¼ tsp black pepper

Directions

i. Put a cooking pan on medium heat.

ii. Add chicken to the skillet after adding a little olive oil to a drizzle.

iii. The chicken should be cooked on both sides until done.

iv. To the pan, add broccoli, bell peppers, and onions.

v. Ensure the vegetables are cooked for another four minutes.

vi.   Add salt and pepper to taste.

Time: 10 minutes

Servings: 1

Nutritional Value

Calories: 350 Fat: 15g Carbohydrates: 10g

Protein: 39gFiber: 4g Sugar: 4g

Veggie Burrito Bowl

Ingredients

- ✓ ½ cup cooked brown rice

- ✓ ¼ cup diced tomatoes

- ✓ 1 tbsp olive oil

- ✓ ¼ tsp sea salt

- ✓ ¼ cup cooked black beans

- ✓ ¼ cup diced bell peppers

- ✓ ¼ cup red onion

- ✓ ¼ tsp black pepper

Directions

i. In a container, combine cooked brown rice, black beans, bell peppers, red onion, and tomatoes.

ii. Dribble olive oil and then add salt, and pepper to the mixture.

iii. Mix until everything is evenly incorporated.

Time: 10 minutes

Servings: 1

Nutritional Value

Calories: 275 Fat: 10g Carbohydrates: 38g

Protein: 8g Fiber: 7g Sugar: 3g

Tuna Salad

Ingredients

- ✓ 4 ounces of canned tuna

- ✓ ¼ cup diced celery

- ✓ 1 tbsp olive oil

- ✓ ¼ tsp sea salt

- ✓ ¼ tsp black pepper

- ✓ ¼ cup diced onion

- ✓ ¼ cup diced tomatoes

Directions

i.   In a container, add tuna, celery, onion, and tomatoes.

ii.   Dribble olive oil and then add salt, and pepper to the mixture.

iii. Mix until everything is evenly incorporated.

Time: 10 minutes

Servings: 1

Nutritional Value

Calories: 250 Fat: 13g Carbohydrates: 10g

Protein: 21g Fiber: 3g Sugar: 5g

Turkey and Quinoa Stuffed Peppers

Ingredients

- ✓ 4 ounces of ground turkey

- ✓ ¼ cup cooked quinoa

- ✓ ¼ cup diced tomatoes

- ✓ 2 tbsp olive oil

- ✓ ¼ tsp of sea salt

- ✓ ¼ tsp black pepper

- ✓ ¼ cup diced bell peppers

- ✓ ¼ cup diced onion

Directions

i.   Preheat oven to 375°F.

ii.   In a container, combine turkey, quinoa, bell peppers, onion, and tomatoes.

iii.   Dribble olive oil and then add salt, and pepper to the mixture.

iv.   Fill the mixture into 4 bell peppers.

v.   Set peppers in a baking dish and bake until peppers are tender, this should take twenty to twenty-five minutes.

Time: 25 minutes

Servings: 4

Nutritional Value

Calories: 250 Fat: 12g Carbohydrates: 21g

Protein: 14g Fiber: 4g Sugar: 5g

Oatmeal

Ingredients

- ✓ ½ cup rolled oats

- ✓ ½ cup unsweetened almond milk

- ✓ ¼ tsp sea salt

- ✓ ¼ cup diced apples

- ✓ ¼ cup diced almonds

- ✓ 1 tbsp honey

Directions

i. In a pan, Add and mix the oats and almond milk.

ii. Cook over medium heat until the oat is done, this should take five to seven minutes.

iii. Add apples, almonds, honey, and salt to the saucepan.

iv.   Stir until everything is evenly incorporated.

Time: 10 minutes

Servings: 1

Nutritional Value

Calories: 350 Fat: 11g Carbohydrates : 50g

Protein: 11g Fiber: 8g Sugar: 15g

Dinner

Mushroom and Black Beans

Ingredients

- ✓ 2 tbsp of extra virgin olive oil

- ✓ 1 cup of diced onion

- ✓ 1 cup of diced carrots

✓ 1 cup of diced celery

✓ 2 minced cloves of garlic

✓ 1 tsp of dried thyme

✓ 2 cups of sliced mushrooms

✓ 2 cups of cooked black beans

✓ ½ cup vegetable stock

✓ Salt

✓ pepper

Directions

i. In a sizable saucepan set over medium heat, preheat the olive oil.

ii. Sauté the onions, carrot, and celery for five minutes while you stir often.

iii. After adding, sauté the garlic and thyme for one minute.

iv. While stirring occasionally, add the mushrooms and simmer for 5 minutes.

v. Add the cooked black beans and vegetable stock, stirring to combine.

vi. Stirring often, bring to a boil, then simmer for fifteen minutes.

vii. Season with salt and pepper to taste.

Time: 25 minutes

Servings: 4

Nutritional Values

Calories: 295 Fat: 7 grams Carbohydrates: 43 grams

Protein: 13 grams Fiber: 11 grams

Rosemary Citrus and Baked Salmon

Ingredients

- ✓ 1 pound salmon fillet

- ✓ 2 tbsp olive oil

- ✓ 2 tbsp lemon juice

- ✓ 2 tbsp orange juice

- ✓ 2 tbsp minced garlic

- ✓ 2 tbsp minced fresh rosemary

- ✓ 1 tsp sea salt

- ✓ 1 tsp freshly ground black pepper

Directions

i.   Preheat oven to 350°F (175°C).

ii.   Place salmon fillet in a greased baking dish.

iii. In a small bowl, combine olive oil, lemon juice, orange juice, garlic, rosemary, salt, and pepper.

iv.   Pour the marinade over the salmon and rub it into the fish to coat.

v.   Bake the salmon until it is well cooked, this should take twenty minutes , then flakes with a fork.

Serving: 4

Nutritional Values

Calories: 203Fat: 10gCarbohydrates: 3g

Protein: 24g

Beef and Barley Stew

Ingredients

- ✓ 2 tbsp of olive oil

- ✓ 1 ¼ pounds of lean beef cubes

- ✓ 1 large onion, chopped

- ✓ 2 cloves of garlic, minced

- ✓ 2 carrots, diced

- ✓ 2 celery stalks, diced

- ✓ 1 cup of pearl barley

- ✓ 2 tablespoons of tomato blend

- ✓ 1 tsp of dried thyme

- ✓ 6 cups of beef broth

- ✓ 2 bay leaves

✓ Salt

✓ pepper

Directions

i.   Add the oil to a pot and heat over medium heat. Once hot, add the beef cubes and cook for 4-5 minutes until lightly browned.

ii.   Add the onion, garlic, carrots, and celery and cook for another 5 minutes until vegetables are softened.

iii.   Add the barley, tomato paste, thyme, beef broth, bay leaves, and salt and pepper to taste.

iv.   Boil for a few minutes, then turn down the heat and simmer for 45 minutes, or until the beef and barley are cooked.

v.   Remove the bay leaves and serve.

Serving: 6

Time: 1hour.

Nutritional Values

Calories: 314 Fat: 8.7gCarbohydrates: 32.3gProtein: 24.3gFiber: 5.3g

Grilled Basil Chicken and Zucchini

Ingredients

- ✓ 2 boneless, skinless chicken breasts

- ✓ 2 tbsp of olive oil

- ✓ 2 cloves of garlic, minced

- ✓ 2 tbsp of fresh basil, chopped

- ✓ 2 medium zucchinis, cut into ½ inch thick slices

- ✓ salt

- ✓ pepper

Directions

i. Preheat the grill to medium-high heat.

ii. Olive oil should be applied to the chicken breasts before seasoning with salt and pepper.

iii. Grill the chicken breasts until they are cooked through and no pink remains, about 10 minutes per side.

iv. In a small bowl, mix together the minced garlic, chopped basil, and a pinch of salt and pepper.

v. Brush the zucchini slices with the garlic and basil mixture.

vi. Place the zucchini slices on the grill and cook for about 4 minutes per side, until tender.

vii.   Serve the grilled basil chicken and zucchini immediately.

Time: 28 minutes

Serving: 2

Nutritional Values

Calories: 214 Fat: 10g Carbohydrates: 5gProtein: 24g

Greek Chicken and Farro Salad

Ingredients

- ✓ 2 cups cooked farro

- ✓ 1 cup cooked chicken, diced

- ✓ ¼ cup feta cheese, crumbled

- ✓ ¼ cup kalamata olives, chopped

- ✓ ¼ cup red onion, diced

- ✓ ¼ cup cucumber, diced

✓ 2 tbsp extra-virgin olive oil

✓ 3 tbsp fresh lemon juice

✓ Salt

✓ Pepper

Directions

i. In a large bowl, combine farro, chicken, feta, olives, red onion, and cucumber.

ii. Whisk the lemon juice, olive oil, pepper, and salt.

iii. Drizzle the mixture over the salad and mix well.

iv. Serve immediately or store in an airtight container in the refrigerator for up to three days.

Time: 10 minutes

Servings: 4

Nutritional Values

Calories: 281Fat: 11gCarbohydrates: 29gProtein: 15gFiber:

5g

Red Curry Shrimps and Cilantro Rice

Ingredients

1 pound of raw, peeled and deveined shrimp

1 cup of long grain white rice

1 tbsp of olive oil

1 tsp of garlic, minced

1 tsp of cumin

1 tsp of red curry paste

¼ tsp of sea salt

¼ cup fresh cilantro, chopped

¼ cup coconut milk

Directions

i. Boil two cups of water in a pot.

ii. Once boiling, add the rice and stir. Lower the heat and ensure the pot is covered. Simmer for 10 minutes.

iii. Heat the olive oil in another pot on medium heat.

iv. Add the minced garlic, cumin, red curry paste, and salt. Cook for 1 minute.

v. Add the shrimp and cook for 3-4 minutes, stirring often.

vi. Add the coconut milk and stir until combined. Cook for an additional 1-2 minutes.

vii. Add the cooked rice and cilantro. Stir to combine. Cook for another 1-2 minutes.

Time: 20 minutes

Servings: 4

Nutritional Values

Calories: 302 kcal Carbohydrates: 33.7 g Fat: 8.5 g

Protein: 23.9 g Sodium: 522 mg Fiber: 2g Sugar: 1g

Creamy Cauliflower Risotto

Ingredients

- ✓ 2 tbsp olive oil

- ✓ 1 diced onion

- ✓ 2 mince garlic

- ✓ 2 cups vegetable broth

- ✓ 1 chopped head cauliflower

- ✓ ¼ cup grated Parmesan cheese

✓ Salt

✓ pepper

Directions

i. The oil should be heated to medium heat. Put in the garlic and onion and sauté for three minutes.

ii. Add the broth and cauliflower to the skillet and bring to a boil.

iii. Reduce the heat to low and simmer for 15 minutes, stirring occasionally, until the cauliflower is softened.

iv. Remove from the heat and stir in the Parmesan cheese. Include salt and pepper as you see appropriate.

Time: 20 minutes

Serving: 4

Nutritional Value

Calories: 164, Fat: 9.5g, Carbohydrates: 13.8g, Protein: 6.9g, Fiber: 3.2g

Baked Cod with Potatoes and Spinach

Ingredients

- ✓ 2 tbsp olive oil
- ✓ 1 diced onion
- ✓ 2 minced cloves garlic
- ✓ 2 cod fillets
- ✓ 2 cups baby spinach
- ✓ 2 potatoes, cut into wedges

✓ ¼ cup grated Parmesan cheese

✓ Salt and pepper to taste.

Directions

i. Preheat the oven to 375 degrees.

ii. The oil should be heated to medium heat. Put in the garlic and onion and sauté for three minutes.

iii. Place the cod in a baking dish and top with the spinach and potatoes.

iv. Dribble with olive oil and top with Parmesan cheese.

v. Bake in preheated oven for 20 minutes, until cod is cooked through, and potatoes are golden brown.

Time: 25 minutes

Serving: 2

Nutritional Values

Calories: 488, Fat: 13.8g, Carbohydrates: 51.4g, Protein: 35.7g, Fiber: 6.4g

Lentil and Kale Soup

Ingredients

- ✓ 2 tbsp olive oil

- ✓ 1 diced onion

- ✓ 2 minced cloves garlic

- ✓ 2 cups vegetable broth

- ✓ 1 cup green lentils

- ✓ 1 cup chopped kale

- ✓ Salt and pepper to taste.

Directions

i. The oil should be heated to medium heat. Put in the garlic and onion and sauté for three minutes.

ii. Add the broth, lentils, and kale to the pot and bring to a boil.

iii. Reduce the heat to low and simmer for 20 minutes, stirring occasionally, until lentils are tender Include salt and pepper as you see appropriate.

Time: 25 minutes

Serving: 4

Nutritional Values

Calories: 160, Fat: 5.4g, Carbohydrates: 20.2g, Protein: 8.1g, Fiber: 5.9g

Grilled Chicken with Roasted Vegetables

Ingredients

- ✓ 2 tablespoons olive oil

- ✓ 2 boneless skinless chicken breasts

- ✓ 2 cups of your favourite vegetables

- ✓ Salt and pepper to taste.

Directions

i. Preheat the grill to medium-high heat.

ii. Apply olive oil to the chicken and add pepper and salt to it.

iii. Grill the chicken for 4 minutes per side, until cooked through.

iv. Sprinkle some olive oil over the vegetables before placing them on a baking sheet.

v. Roast in preheated oven for 20 minutes, until vegetables are tender.

vi. Serve the chicken with the roasted vegetables.

Time: 25

Serving: 2

Nutritional Values

Calories: 382, Fat: 12.4g, Carbohydrates: 19.2g, Protein: 43.7g, Fiber: 4.9g

Turkey Burgers with Zucchini Fries

Ingredients

- ✓ 1 pound ground turkey

- ✓ ¼ cup breadcrumbs

- ✓ 2 mincedcloves garlic

- ✓ ¼ cup diced onion

✓ 1 egg

✓ 2 medium zucchini, cut into strips

✓ 2 tbsp olive oil

✓ Salt and pepper to taste.

Directions

i.   In a large bowl, mix together the turkey, breadcrumbs, garlic, onion, and egg. Form into four patties.

ii. The oil should be heated to medium heat. Add the zucchini strips and cook for 10 minutes, until golden brown.

iii. In the same skillet, add the turkey patties and cook for 5 minutes per side, until cooked through.

iv.   Serve the turkey burgers with the zucchini fries.

Time: 25 minutes

Serving: 4

Nutritional Values

Calories: 326, Fat: 12.3g, Carbohydrates: 15.3g, Protein: 37.7g, Fiber: 2.8g

Snacks

Apple Slices with Peanut Butter

Ingredients

✓ 2 apples

✓ 2 tbsp of natural peanut butter

Directions

i. Slice the apples into thin wedges.

ii. Onto the apple slices, apply the peanut butter.

Time: 10 minutes

Serving: 2

Nutritional Values

Calories: 128 Protein: 4g Fat: 6g

Carbohydrates: 18g Fiber: 4g

Trail Mix

Ingredients

- ✓ ¼ cup of almonds

- ✓ ¼ cup of dried cranberries

- ✓ ¼ cup of pumpkin seeds

✓ ¼ cup of dark chocolate chips

Directions

i.   In a dish, put all the ingredients.

ii.   Mix the ingredients together.

Time: 10 minutes

Serving: 1

Nutritional Values

Calories: 244 Protein: 8g Fat: 16g Carbohydrates: 19g

Fiber: 5g

Cottage Cheese and Berries

Ingredients

✓ ½ cup cottage cheese

✓ ¼ cup blueberries

✓ ¼ cup raspberries

Directions

i. Measure out the cottage cheese and place it in a bowl.

ii. Add the blueberries and raspberries to the cottage cheese and mix together.

Time: 5 minutes

Serving: 1

Nutritional Values

Calories: 137 Protein: 15g Fat: 2g Carbohydrates: 12g Fiber: 2g

Banana Smoothie

Ingredients

- ✓ 1 banana

- ✓ ½ cup plain Greek yogurt

- ✓ ½ cup almond milk

- ✓ 1 tbsp of honey

Directions

i. Put the banana in the processor after peeling it.

ii. Add the yogurt, almond milk, and honey to the blender and blend until smooth.

Time: 5 minutes

Serving: 1

Nutritional Values

Calories: 177 Prothein: 9g Fat: 2g Carbohydrates: 31g

Fiber: 2g

Baked Sweet Potato Fries

Ingredients

- ✓ 2 sweet potatoes

- ✓ 2 tbsp olive oil

- ✓ Salt

- ✓ pepper

Directions

i. Preheat oven to 350°F.

ii. Cut the sweet potatoes into thin strips.

iii. Add salt and pepper to the sweet potatoes after rubbing them with olive oil.

iv. Bake the sweet potatoes for 20 minutes, turning them over halfway through.

Time: 25 minutes

Serving: 2

Nutritional Values

Calories: 193 Protein: 3g Fat: 10g Carbohydrates: 25g

Fiber: 4g

Desserts

Oatmeal Chocolate Chip Cookies

Ingredients

- ✓ 1 cup rolled oats.

- ✓ 1 cup whole wheat flour

- ✓ ½ cup dark chocolate chips

- ✓ 1/3 cup coconut oil

✓ 1/3 cup honey

✓ 1 teaspoon baking powder

✓ ½ tsp baking soda

✓ 1/2 tsp salt

Directions

i.   Preheat the oven to 350°F.

ii.   In a large bowl, mix together rolled oats, whole wheat flour, dark chocolate chips, baking powder, baking soda, and salt.

iii.   In a separate bowl, mix together the coconut oil d honey until blended.

iv.   Put all the wet ingredients together with the dry ingredients and stir until well incorporated.

v.   Line a baking sheet with parchment paper and drop the cookie dough onto the baking sheet.

vi.   Put in the oven till the edges are lightly golden, this should take 10-12 minutes.

vii. Take it out of the oven then serve after it has cool down.

Time: 25 minutes

Servings: 12

Nutritional value

110 calories, 5g fat, 17g carbs, 2g protein

Coconut Chia Pudding

Ingredients

- ✓ 1 cup full-fat coconut milk

- ✓ 2 tbsp chia seeds

- ✓ 2 tbsp honey

- ✓ ½ tsp vanilla extract

Directions

i. Mix the coconut milk, chia seeds, honey, and vanilla extract in a mixing container.

ii. For at least four hours or overnight, cover the container and store it in the refrigerator. Stir the chia pudding before serving.

Time: 4 hours

Servings: 2

Nutritional value

190 calories, 14g fat, 14g carbs, 4g protein

Baked Apples

Ingredients

- ✓ 4 sliced apples
- ✓ ¼ cup raisins
- ✓ ¼ cup chopped walnuts, chopped
- ✓ 1 tsp ground cinnamon
- ✓ 1 tbsp coconut oil
- ✓ 2 tbsp honey

Directions

i. Preheat the oven to 375°F.

ii. Apple slices should be put in a baking dish.

iii. In a small bowl, mix together the raisins, walnuts, and cinnamon.

iv.   Sprinkle the mixture over the apples and drizzle with coconut oil and honey.

v.   The apples should be baked for 20 to 25 minutes, or until they are soft.

Time: 25 minutes

Servings: 4

Nutritional value

110 calories, 5g fat, 16g carbs, 2g protein

Banana Oatmeal Pancakes

Ingredients

- ✓ 1 large, mashed banana

- ✓ ½ cup rolled oats

- ✓ ¼ tsp baking powder

- ✓ ¼ tsp baking soda

✓ ¼ tsp ground cinnamon

✓ ¼ cup almond milk

✓ 2 tbsp honey

Directions

i. Mash the banana in a mixing bowl until it is nearly smooth.

ii. Add the rolled oats, baking powder, baking soda, ground cinnamon, almond milk, and honey. Mix until combined.

iii. Grease a nonstick skillet with coconut oil and cook over medium heat.

iv. 1/4 cup of the batter should be dropped onto the skillet, and it should fry for 2–3 minutes, or till golden brown.

v.   Cook the other side for 2 more minutes or until golden.

vi.   Serve with your favorite toppings.

Time: 10 minutes

Servings: 2

Nutritional value

210 calories, 6g fat, 36g carbs, 5g protein

Baked Pears with Walnuts

Ingredients

- ✓ 2 pears, sliced

- ✓ ¼ cup chopped walnuts

- ✓ 1 tsp ground cinnamon

- ✓ 2 tbsp honey

Directions

i.   Preheat the oven to 375°F.

ii.   Slices of pears should be put on a baking dish.

iii.   Sprinkle with the walnuts and cinnamon.

iv.   Drizzle with honey.

v.   Bake the pears for 20 to 25 minutes, or until they are tender.

Time: 25 minutes

Servings: 2

Nutritional value

130 calories, 5g fat, 20g carbs, 2g protein

Appetizer

Tomato and Basil Bruschetta

Ingredients

- ✓ 2 tomatoes, diced

- ✓ 2 cloves garlic, minced

- ✓ 2 tbsp extra-virgin olive oil

- ✓ 2 tbsp fresh basil, chopped

- ✓ 2 tbsp balsamic vinegar

- ✓ 1 loaf of French bread, sliced

Directions

i. Preheat oven to 350°F.

ii. In a medium bowl, combine tomatoes, garlic, olive oil, basil, and balsamic vinegar.

iii.   Place bread slices on a baking sheet.

iv.   Top each slice with bruschetta mixture.

v.   Bake in preheated oven for 10 minutes, or until
bread is toasted.

Time: 15 minutes

Serving: 4

Nutritional Values

Calories: 175; Fat: 8g; Carbohydrates: 20g; Protein: 4g;
Fiber: 2

Avocado Cucumber Bites

Ingredients

- ✓ 1 avocado, mashed

- ✓ 1 cucumber, diced

- ✓ 2 tbsp lemon juice

- ✓ 2 tbsp fresh parsley, chopped

- ✓ ½ tsp garlic powder

- ✓ ¼ tsp sea salt

Directions

i.   In a medium bowl, combine mashed avocado,

ii. cucumber, lemon juice, parsley, garlic powder, and salt.

iii. Mix until well combined.

iv. Spoon mixture onto cucumber slices and serve.

Time: 10 minutes

Serving: 4

Nutritional Values

Calories: 67; Fat: 5g; Carbohydrates: 5g; Protein: 1g; Fiber: 2g

Roasted Sweet Potato Rounds

Ingredients

- ✓ 2 sweet potatoes, sliced into 1/2-inch rounds

- ✓ 2 tbsp olive oil

- ✓ 1 tsp garlic powder

- ✓ 1 tsp smoked paprika

- ✓ ½ tsp sea salt

Directions

i. Preheat oven to 375°F.

ii. In a large bowl, mix together sweet potato rounds, olive oil, garlic powder, smoked paprika, and sea salt.

iii. Spread sweet potato rounds on a baking sheet and bake for 25 minutes, or until potatoes are tender.

iv.   Serve warm.

Time: 30 minutes

Serving: 4

Nutritional Values

Calories: 145; Fat: 7g; Carbohydrates: 18g; Protein: 2g; Fiber: 3g

Spicy Roasted Chickpeas

Ingredients

- ✓ 1 can chickpeas, drained and rinsed
- ✓ 1 tbsp olive oil
- ✓ 1 tsp cumin
- ✓ 1 tsp chili powder
- ✓ ½ tsp garlic powder
- ✓ ½ tsp sea salt

Directions

i. Preheat oven to 375°F.

ii. In a medium bowl, combine chickpeas, olive oil, cumin, chili powder, garlic powder, and salt.

iii. On a baking sheet, spread out the chickpeas and bake for 25 minutes, or until golden brown.

iv. Serve warm.

Time: 30 minutes

Serving: 4

Nutritional Values

Calories: 145; Fat: 4g; Carbohydrates: 20g; Protein: 5g; Fiber: 5g

CONCLUSION

The Endomorph Diet Cookbook has provided readers with an extensive variety of recipes that are specifically tailored to the endomorph body type. The recipes are easy to follow and provide a wide range of flavors and ingredients that can be used to create delicious and nutritious meals. With a focus on healthy fats and proteins, endomorphs can enjoy a variety of meals that are both tasty and beneficial to their health.

Additionally, the recipes provide easy-to-follow instructions and a wide range of flavors and ingredients that can be used to create nutritious and delicious meals. With this cookbook, endomorphs can enjoy meals that are both tasty and beneficial to their health.

You may achieve your fitness objectives while losing those extra pounds by understanding your body type, especially if you are an endomorph and adhering to the endomorph diet

plan's rules. Eat as advised by your doctor, chew your food

thoroughly and do not live a sedentary life.

www.ingramcontent.com/pod-product-compliance
Lightning Source LLC
Chambersburg PA
CBHW051216250726

48655CB00006B/2438